Attachment and Suicidality in Youth

About the Author
David Cawthorpe, PhD

Dr. Cawthorpe completed a Master's degree in biochemical mechanisms of learning and memory and a Doctoral degree in human attachment focusing on the relationship of attachment and depression in a clinical sample. He has published extensively in the areas of epidemiology and psychiatric medicine. Dr. Cawthorpe has developed three electronic records with embedded clinical screening and patient-centered outcome measurement, sensitive enough to measure the effects of clinical teaching in the community in terms of the post-training changes in the quality and quantity of subsequent referrals to centralized regional health services. He is currently an adjunct professor in the Faculty of Medicine at the University of Calgary.

©DavidCawthorpe

All rights reserved

ISBN: 9781720221579

Table of Contents

Forward 1
Introduction 5
Attachment Theory - An Overview 9
Attachment Behavior 15
Working Models 21
Factors related to Suicidal Behavior and Suicide 35
   Demographic Approaches 35
   Attempters and Completers 36
   Mental Disorders and Genetic Factors 37
   Psychological Factors and Social Isolation 38
   Developmental Factors 42
   Family Factors 44
Attachment Theory and Suicide 49
Sex Differences and Attachment 57
Summary 63
References 67

Forward

Suicidal behaviour in adolescence remains a major public health issue (Lachal, Moro, & Spodenkiewicz, 2018). Attempters that repeated attempt suicide appear to have more psychological features impairing emotional stability which may be related to insecure anxious attachment (Pennel, Quesada, & Dematteis, 2018). Insecure attachment is associated with suicidal behavior (Adam, Sheldon-Keller, & West, 1996) and has a bearing on therapeutic intervention (Li et al., 2017). Study focusing on attachment aims to develop a theoretical framework for the role played by connectedness (attachment) in relation to suicide (Aherne, Coughlan, & Surgenor, 2018). For example, within the construct of insecure attachment, the personality dimensions of self-criticism rather than dependency has been identified as risk factors for suicide in adolescents (Falgares et al., 2017). In clinical samples, negative expectancies for caregiver availability have been associated both with attachment insecurity and with the intensity of adolescents' suicidal ideation (Zisk, Abbott, Ewing, Diamond, & Kobak, 2017). Theories of suicidal behavior suggest that suicidality arises from the disruption of interpersonal relationships (Sheftall, Mathias, Furr, & Dougherty, 2013). Much remains to be learned about the mechanisms that account for the relationship between attachment styles and severity of suicidal ideation (Zisk et al., 2017).

One thing is certain. For better or worse, the personality of every human being emerges from a primary attachment relationship. The pathway to suicidality is complex and multiform and the quality of family relationships is one key factor modulating the trajectory of development toward or away from suicidality (Bowlby, 1977; Lavigne et al., 2016).

Introduction

The purpose of this book is to describe the relevance of attachment theory to suicidal behavior. Suicidal behavior and completed suicide are complex phenomena influenced by multiple factors that vary across the life cycle. While no model yet developed adequately predicts whether an individual will engage in suicidal behavior or commit suicide, research into the factors related to increased risk point to the importance of family factors. For example, poor family relationships are a common gateway leading to increased risk of suicidal behaviors and suicide (Adam, 1990). Attachment theory offers both a conceptual framework and an empirical basis for understanding the development of family relationships, in particular child-parent attachment relationships and their contribution to individual psychosocial adaptation across the life cycle. It follows that attachment theory can provide insight into the family relationships that protect an individual from adversity or increase the risk for suicidal behavior and suicide (Adam, 1990, 1994; Adam, Sheldon-Keller & West, 1996).

Research across several domains seeks to account for both suicidal behavior and suicide. For example, demographic approaches to suicidal behavior and completed suicide indicate differences for males and females and variations across stages of the life cycle. This book begins with an overview of first, attachment theory and second, the range of factors related to increased risk of suicidal behavior and suicide. In the last section, the relevance of attachment theory to suicidal behavior is brought into focus upon review of published evidence. In summary, a promising area of intervention is outlined.

Attachment Theory - An Overview

Attachment theory integrates ethological and psychoanalytic principles in describing the origins and growth of human personality (Bowlby, 1969, 1973, 1980). Both ethological and psychoanalytic perspectives view the child-parent relationship as central to the developmental process. Within attachment theory, the psychoanalytic perspective provides a framework for understanding personality development and the emergence of psychopathology in terms of how the relationship between a parent's own past experiences and current state of mind influences the personality development of his or her children (Main, Kaplan & Cassidy, 1985; Ricks, 1985).

From ethology comes the understanding that similar to other altricial species, there is a biological mandate conferred by evolution for humans to protect and care for their young, thereby promoting survival, and ultimately perpetuation of the species. An infant is born with a *biological expectation* that a caregiver is present. An infant enters the world prepared for care, with well-developed senses and a complex set of reflexes, expressive behaviors and affects that facilitate immediate survival (Hoffer, 1981). Infant behavior complements caregiving behavior. The rhythm and contingency of this interaction serve to regulate the infant's inner world, and contribute to the development in the infant of awareness, discernment, emotional regulation and the attachment relationship (Dodge, 1991; Stern, 1985).

Protection and personality growth occur in the context of the child-caregiver relationship (George, 1994). Protection represents the continuous biological function of the attachment relationship. This function is independent of individual characteristics or levels of development. Parental caregiving behavior and a child's attachment behavior vary according to the level of development and individual characteristics, yet these behaviors are organized around providing protection through seeking proximity in the face of real or perceived threat or danger. For example, in the face of perceived threat (e.g. a stranger), a baby will crawl to a parent to be picked up and reassured, whereas an older child may simply move closer to his caregiver or establish eye contact. Alternatively, a parent may pick up and carry his or her small child when in a crowd, or seek to hold an older child's hand in order to prevent the danger of separation (George, 1994).

Attachment Behavior

Ainsworth was the first to systematically categorize the various patterns of attachment behavior observed in infants using an experimental method known as the *strange situation* that involved a number of structured separations and reunions with the caregiver (Ainsworth et al., 1978). Several categories of behavior are currently described in the literature. The infant behavior categories originally described by Ainsworth et al. (1978) were termed secure, ambivalent and avoidant. Upon reunion in the *strange* situation, secure infants seek proximity and physical contact with the parent and are easily comforted upon reunion (Ainsworth et al. 1978). This optimal behavior, associated with parents who promptly and successfully interact providing protection and care, is termed a primary attachment strategy (Main, 1989).

Avoidant infants respond by ignoring or actively avoiding parents upon reunion, while ambivalent infants seek proximity and physical contact, yet appear unsatisfied, remaining angry and upset (Ainsworth et al. 1978). Ambivalent and avoidant attachment strategies are termed secondary, in that protection is not unconditional (Main, 1989). The child is not secure in his or her relationship with the parent and develops secondary strategies to meet attachment needs. Avoidant infants remain in only relative proximity to the care-giver. They maintain proximity and achieve protection through deactivating attachment behavior, though their internal stress remains high.

The development of avoidant behavior is associated with consistent parental rejection of the infant's primary attachment behavior.

Ambivalent infants develop in the opposite direction, their attachment behaviors are amplified, and they seek proximity without parental contact serving to provide the comfort and reassurance that terminates their attachment behavior (Marvin, 1977). Their anxiety, anger and resistance persist in the face of their caregivers' unsuccessful attempts to provide comfort. Ambivalence (proximity-seeking with concomitant anger and resistance) is associated with inconsistent parental responsiveness and care.

Secure, avoidant and ambivalent attachment behaviors represent organized strategies reflecting a relatively coherent set of rules based upon past experiences with caregivers that guide behavior upon perception of danger or threat.

Researchers studying high risk samples recently identified an additional group of infants, termed disorganized. Disorganized infants exhibit atypical attachment behavior (Crittenden, 1988; Main & Solomon, 1990). Unlike the other categories, the behavior of disorganized infants does not appear organized or adaptive in that they fail to achieve proximity or protection. Rather, upon reunion in the strange situation, they appear fearful or freeze, exhibiting unusual movements suggesting inner conflict as though the care-giver is perceived as both a source of protection and potential harm (Main & Hesse, 1990; Cicchetti & Toth, 1995). Additionally, some investigators pose that disorganization may also result when an infant perceives his source of protection or caregiver as overwhelmed by fear (George, 1994).

Working Models

In addition to physical safety, nurturance and succor, care-givers' affective and behavioral responses to a child provide the child with an inner sense of security and expectations regarding the future availability and responsiveness of the care-giver. Observations from the *strange situation* support this view. To account for complex developmental changes and variations in attachment behaviors based upon experiences with care-givers, Bowlby (1969/1982, 1973) proposed that a child's attachment behavior was guided by the development of cognitive representations or working models of the self and the attachment figure (or care-giver).

Main, Kaplan, & Cassidy (1985) proposed that working models of the self and the attachment figure begin to develop during the first few months of life. A child's patterns of response or attachment behavior tend to stabilize, and like the working model, reflect variations in the quality of actual interactions and experiences with the caregiver. (Ainsworth, Blehar, Waters, & Wall, 1978; Radke-Yarrow, Cummings, Kuczynski, & Chapman, 1985). Infants and children, like adults, use their working models to appraise attachment-related information and guide their behavior (Bowlby, 1969/1982, 1973).

During the pre-school years, in addition to an increasing awareness of himself and his own needs, a child more or less comes to better appreciate the goals, feelings and state of mind of the caregiver. The child's volition and *novel* self-other awareness begin what Bowlby termed the *goal-directed partnership*. During this period the child, of himself, becomes a great and more focused force in the child-parent relationship (George, 1994); the child and parent more actively recognize differences in their plans. They are perhaps better able to negotiate and pursue their goals, depending upon how they have come to relate, and depending upon the working models of the child and parent, and in particular the defensive mechanisms carried forward by the parent (Bowlby, 1973; Marvin & Greenberg, 1982; Main, Kaplan & Cassidy, 1985). This shift in the perspective of the child reflects a developing agency of self and an understanding that the self and the attachment figure are separate (West, 1995). The child comes to reflect more upon his working model, rather than relying on the actual presence of his caregiver (Crittenden & Ainsworth, 1989). With this the stage is set for attachment across the life span (George, 1994).

Across development, the working model continues to accommodate new experiences with the caregiver, and those arising from the developing self-reflective and cognitive abilities of the child (e.g. the ability to think about the attachment relationship; George, 1994). However, such accommodation may be constrained by a number of factors that guide the development and function of the working model (Bretherton, 1985; Main Kaplan & Cassidy, 1985; Sroufe & Fleeson, 1986). For instance, previous experiences with caregivers influence the responses of the individual in the present. In other words, current thought about attachment figures and responses to them are influenced by the working model carried forward from the past.

The model carried forward is determined by the perceptual record of the temporal, spatial, interactive and affective aspects of past experiences. The abstraction and organization of such collective perceptual records into mental representations is explained in terms of schemas, scripts or memories. Further, how such memory-based structures are made available and constitute working models gives rise to the operation of rules or governing cognitive structures. For example, working models are thought to involve defensive processes that influence both how an individual perceives the present situation, what he or she remembers about past attachment related experiences and ultimately how he or she will respond (Bowlby, 1973; Main et al. 1985). Such processes may operate outside the conscious awareness of an individual. Current theory holds cognitive and affective systems to be thoroughly interdependent, integrated systems that order the mental contents and guide responses based upon the perception of internal and external stimuli (Dodge, 1991). This view is more in keeping with current discussions of physiological structure-function relationships within the tissue of the brain (Tucker, 1992; Dodge, 1991; Edelman, 1987; Ono, et al. 1993).

Fonagy and others (1991) drew upon the work of Fraiberg (1975) to examine what mechanisms determine whether or not the conflicted past of a parent will repeat itself in the child. Like Fraiberg, they concluded that accounting for such inter-generational transmission lies in an understanding of the defenses (such as denial of affect) used by a parent to cope with a difficult past and their capacity for self-reflection; the capacity to reflect upon mental contents and function in oneself and others. They trace the natural development of self-reflective capacity from early childhood and note that this capacity is dramatically constrained in serious pathological disorders, such as borderline personality disorder (Fonagy et al., 1993).

The internal working models grow in capacity and complexity with development and form the basis for the individual to maintain a felt sense of security in the absence of their attachment figure. As the parent provided a secure base with their physical presence from which the infant explored early in development, an inner sense of security facilitates within the individual the ability to focus upon activities and pursue goals unrelated to attachment (West & Keller, 1994).

Increasing functional complexity of mental representation facilitates dealing with conflicting feelings about experiences with the attachment figure (West & Keller, 1994). Such information may be partitioned or compartmentalized and possibly restricted from consciousness, forming a basis for the maintenance of multiple working models (Main, Kaplan & Cassidy, 1985). West and

Keller (1994) suggest that when representations are thus separated, there ensues a limited capacity for integration and self-reflection.

In the presence of a limited capacity for self-reflection, an individual's adaptive ability is constrained. Fewer adaptive choices are available together with a constricted ability to reflect upon, regulate or integrate inner emotional experiences. Such an individual depends more on the external environment for emotional regulation and guidance, leaving him or her more prone and vulnerable to relational difficulties.

West & Keller (1994) recast the definition of working models by integrating a contemporary model of functional memory (Edelman, 1994). Affects or emotions are the driving forces in the formation, maintenance and activation of internal working models. Accordingly, an individual is emotionally primed by past experiences with attachment figures to respond to behavioral and affect cues that "reactivate in the present the affect category established in the past" (p. 64; West & Keller, 1994).

Emotional regulation, insecure attachment, and behavioral problems that emerge in early childhood appear to be maintained, or modified, along the path to adolescence through ongoing, if not repetitive transactions within primary family relationships. Such transactions serve to facilitate or prevent adaptive retranscription of the individual's internal working model. Emotional regulation and autonomy come to be mastered through the contingency of parental responsiveness and in particular the cogent expression of affective meaning and value.

Main & Goldwyn (1991) provided empirical evidence regarding the nature of the internal working models of adults. This evidence comes from the adult attachment interview (AAI); a structured interview that evaluates an individual's current state of mind with respect to attachment. The content and coherency of discourse that an individual can maintain and reflect upon in communicating about their current and past attachment experiences reveals this current state of mind.

The interview reveals four categories of adult coherency of mind with respect to attachment that parallel the behavioral categories observed in infants; these are termed autonomous (secure), dismissing (avoidant), preoccupied (ambivalent) and unresolved with respect to trauma (disorganized): 1) Autonomous/secure adults attend to the interview and respond in an organized, coherent manner with memories of their attachment experiences that support their current evaluations, whether these are good and/or bad. 2) Preoccupied/ambivalent adults tend to respond at length to interview questions indicating their degree of involvement with their attachment experiences. They respond in either angry and/or passive ways that are characteristically incoherent.

3) Dismissing/avoidant adults devalue, idealize or normalize attachment relationships. Their responses are often terse and brief. They distance emotional content

and render the influence of their attachment experiences to a minimum. 4) Unresolved/disorganized individuals tend not to maintain coherent communication, especially when recounting traumatic experiences such as loss or abuse. They present evidence of unusual beliefs about their experiences and lapses in thinking and logic.

Traditionally, the relationship of attachment status, childhood adjustment problems and the development of psychopathology was conceptualized along one axis, the secure-insecure continuum (Sroufe, 1983, 1988). Recently, evidence suggests that while insecure infants and children (ambivalent and avoidant) show somewhat less optimal social adjustment, they are able to adapt to their parents and organize strategies around meeting attachment needs. Those classified as disorganized are now thought to be most prone to later development of more serious psychiatric problems (Cicchetti & Toth, 1995; Adam, Sheldon-Keller & West, 1995). Based on work with high risk groups of children, attachment researchers currently conceptualize the relationship of attachment status and psychopathology along two axes, a secure-insecure axis and an organized-disorganized axis (George, 1994). From this formulation of the relationship between attachment and psychopathology, it follows that those who are unresolved with respect to past trauma are at greatest risk for suicidal behavior.

Factors related to Suicidal Behavior and Suicide

Demographic Approaches

Suicide, the willful ending of one's own existence, is most often found in association with mental and/or physical illness (Bongar, 1992). Suicide is well studied in terms of demographic disparities that arise between variables such as sex and age (Shneidman, 1992). For example, men complete suicide more often than women. With respect to age, the elderly have the highest rate of suicide, though this has decreased over time, while the rate for adolescents increased threefold between 1950 and 1980. The list goes on to include disparities in locations (countries, states, cities) and disparities in census variables (occupation and socioeconomic status). Generally, suicide and attempted suicide are associated with poor living circumstances, loss of socio-economic status and other indices of social disorganization, such as transience, unemployment, etc. (reviewed by Adam, 1990). Demographic approaches to suicide provide insight into high risk groups and the changes in the profiles of such groups over time (Vaillant & Blumenthal, 1990).

Attempters and Completers

There are differences between those who attempt suicide and those who complete suicide across demographic variables, such as sex, ethnicity and age (Clark & Fawcett, 1992; Vaillant &

Blumenthal, 1990). For instance, whites are more likely to commit suicide than non-whites, whereas race and ethnicity do not appear to distinguish non-fatal suicide attempters. As opposed to completed suicide, females are more likely to attempt suicide than males. Similarly, with respect to age, those under forty-five years of age are more likely to attempt suicide than older persons, and people separated or divorced are more likely to attempt than those who are espoused.

Mental Disorders and Genetic Factors

The occurrence of suicide in the absence of a mental disorder is rare. Studies in the last four decades indicate that major depression and/or alcoholism are most commonly found in association with suicide, followed by categories of mental disorder, such as cycling bipolar affective disorder and schizophrenia (Clark & Fawcett, 1992). While there is good evidence that affective disorders and schizophrenia have a genetic basis, a similar genetically based component for suicide has not been demonstrated (Lester, 1988; Seymour, 1990).

Psychological Factors and Social Isolation

The demographic approach provides little information about the dynamic between psychopathology, suicidal behavior and completed suicide (Bongar, 1992). On the other hand, approaches that take into account clinical, case-study observations, personal documents and individual history provide a rich source of information regarding psychological factors common to suicidality. For example, according to Shneidman (1992), suicide is a solution by which to escape intolerable, psychological pain that results from the experience of unbearable circumstances. The circumstances that give rise to such pain, and the unwillingness to bear it, are variable, yet tend to involve the frustration of personal needs such as the need for nurturance and succor. Frustration and psychological pain are accompanied by a sense of futility, ambivalence, helplessness and hopelessness, together with a constrained view of the solutions available to tolerate and resolve both inner and outer conflicts. Furthermore, while suicide is a final act, the life-long patterns of coping employed by suicidal individuals tend to be consistent (Shneidman, 1992). In other words, suicidal individuals are thought to consistently behave in ways that validate their viewpoint, undermine potentially supportive relationships and contribute to their social isolation.

In much the same way that Brown and Harris (1978) described the pathway to depression, factors such as negative life events, social disorganization (e.g. transience and unemployment) and personal difficulties (e.g. divorce or separation) interact with individual proclivities leading to real or perceived social isolation and increased risk of suicidal behavior (Adam, 1990). Attempters and completers may differ in their degree of social isolation. For example, attempters are more socially engaged and often appeal to others in their social environment, whereas completers rarely do, perhaps reflecting a greater degree of social isolation (Adam, 1990).

Developmental Factors

Development and developmental decline may contribute to both protection and risk of suicide at different stages of the life cycle. Completed suicide before puberty is rare, yet it is cited as the seventh leading cause of death in five to fourteen year olds, and is more common in boys than girls (National Center for Health Statistics, 1990; Sokol & Pfeffer, 1992). In contrast, suicide is the third leading cause of death in adolescents, and again it is more common in males (Sokol & Pfeffer, 1992). Protective developmental factors that in part account for the differences between children and adolescents may include the lack of advanced cognitive and physical abilities in children thought necessary to conceptualize the act of suicide, maintain a plan and carry it out (Pfeffer & Sokol, 1992).

During middle and late adolescence, the rate of suicide and attempted suicide rises dramatically, concomitant with developing cognitive abilities. Cognitive development may account in part for increased vulnerability to depression and suicidality (Vaillant & Blumenthal, 1990). During adolescence there is increased exposure to risk factors such as drugs, alcohol and weapons. A lack of the experience necessary to develop and exercise strategies for dealing with such dangers combined with the lack of a protective environment leaves a young person more vulnerable at this stage of development (Vaillant & Blumenthal, 1990).

With old age and developmental decline suicide rates rise again. Old age is associated mental and physical impairment and can result in increased hopelessness, social isolation and despair, thereby increasing the risk of suicide (Vaillant & Blumenthal, 1990).

Family Factors

As noted above, children are thought to be less susceptible to the hopelessness and despair that accompany suicidality and depression. While this may account in part for decreased rates of depression and suicidality, these phenomena are well documented in children, though the forms of expression appear more transient and less abstract than in adults (Sokol & Pfeffer, 1992).

A variety of mental problems are associated with increased risk of suicidality. Antisocial behavior, conduct disorder and impulse control problems are risk factors; children and adolescents with co-morbid affective disorder are at particular risk (Alessi et al., 1984). Longitudinal studies indicated in children and adolescents that early onset of affective disorder, co-morbidity with other disorders, and recurrent depressive episodes are related to increased rates of suicidal behavior (Kovacs et al. 1993; Rao et al. 1993). Membership in a high risk peer group, together with drug and alcohol abuse increases the risk for suicidal behavior (Pfeffer, et al. 1988). Children of abusive, neglectful parents or parents with depression, substance abuse problems or suicidal behaviors are also at increased risk of suicidal behavior (Sokol & Pfeffer, 1992).

Factors such as child psychopathology, substance abuse problems, parental psychopathology, poor parenting, abuse and neglect rarely operate in isolation. This places the nexus for developing suicidal propensities within a family context. For example, some children and adolescents who face similar painful circumstances and stresses do not become depressed and suicidal. The resilience and adaptive capacity of such children is related to the presence of a number of protective factors; these include external supports and resources that center around family cohesion and warmth with the absence of discord and neglect, together with an inner sense of self-esteem, autonomy and control (Garmezy, 1985; Rutter, 1989).

Attachment Theory and Suicide

A chaotic home-life, adverse circumstances, disruption and stresses within a family lead to poor parental care and increase the likelihood that parents are unavailable, unresponsive or abusive. These factors predispose a child to suicidality and mental disorder. In addition, early loss of a parent has been cited as an important factor in the etiology of depression and suicidal behavior, though it is less well understood in those who complete suicide (Adam, 1990). However, Adam (1990) suggests that when early loss of a parent makes its effect known in the form of later psychopathology or suicidality, the loss is more an indication of the long-term disruption of family stability and failure to resolve the loss, than an effect of the loss itself. This is the case whether loss is from death, divorce or adoption (Adam, 1994).

It is mistaken to think that early experiences alone lead directly to either mental disorder, suicidality or completed suicide. It is more likely that early experiences mediated by internal working models lead to the development of enduring personality characteristics and coping strategies through ongoing interactions and situations (Adam, 1990).

Ongoing adversity operates to undermine opportunities for the child to make sense of what happens or resolve his experience with caregivers or re-transcribe his working model. Under adverse circumstances the child lives in fear and uncertainty; unable to form a stable, adaptable set of expectations the child has no means to predict either parental behavior or his own resulting inner state. Attachment theory's proponents argue that a child's immediate and specific responses to conflict and the emotional unavailability of the parent result in a patterning of behavior and emotional responses that are persistent, as reflected in the behavior of the very young and in the working models of older children and adults (Ainsworth et al. 1978; George, 1994; Main, Kaplan & Cassidy, 1985; Main & Solomon, 1990, Main 1989, 1990; Sroufe & Waters, 1977). In addition to their relationship with the development of insecure attachment, emotional and behavior problems in children, parental unavailability and emotional unresponsiveness are factors also linked to parental mental disorder, substance abuse or family adversity arising from separation or loss from death or divorce (Cicchetti & Toth, 1993, 1995; Radke-Yarrow, Cummings, Kuczynski, & Chapman, 1985; Zahn-Waxler, Cummings, Iannotti, & Radke-Yarrow, 1984).

An adverse childhood often leaves an individual with persistent immature, hostile and impulsive characteristics that fail to regulate an individual's inner experience, but rather serve to undermine supportive relationships leading to increased social isolation (Adam, 1990). According to the attachment theory, working models are the agents mediating past experiences and the personality characteristics that predispose an individual to mental disorder and suicidality (Adam, 1990).

Those who commit or attempt suicide usually experience conflict in close personal relationships shortly prior to the event (Adam, 1990, 1994). Such conflict often takes the form of threatened separations and quarrels with parents, siblings, peers, opposite sexed friends, lovers or spouses. The gravity of family conflict is found in some instances to be extreme, with profound rejection and hostility directed at the suicidal member (Adam, 1990). The personal difficulties of suicidal individuals appear to be long-standing in nature, rather than transient. Adam (1994) proposed that suicide is an extreme attachment behavior that expresses distress and anger toward an unavailable or unresponsive attachment figure in a failed attempt to achieve proximity, security and comfort. This is reminiscent of the behavior of the ambivalent child, who is unable to find comfort and security in the arms of the caregiver.

De Jong (1992) examined the history of suicidality in a non-clinical sample of college students and found that suicidality was related to greater insecurity of attachment to parents. Similarly, Adam, Sheldon-Keller and West (1996) were able to confirm the formulation that suicidal behavior is an extreme form of attachment behavior. In a retrospective case-comparison study, these researchers found that those exhibiting suicidal behavior and ideation were differentiated from those in a clinical comparison group with no history of suicidality using the Adult Attachment Interview (Main & Goldwyn, 1991).

Consistent with other literature, older females in the sample had a greater frequency of past suicidality (Adam, Sheldon-Keller & West, 1996). Suicidal individuals of both sexes were most frequently classified as preoccupied and unresolved/disorganized (unresolved with respect to attachment experiences). The adult attachment interview taps an individual's current state of mind with respect to attachment and hence indicates the current influence of past events. The suicidal case group and non-suicidal, clinical comparison group did not differ with respect to their exposure to trauma, but the suicidal group differed in being unresolved with respect to past trauma.

The results of the Adam, West and Keller (1996) study support the view that two axes of attachment classification are important with respect to suicidality. Risk of suicidality as determined by attachment status is related to both a secure-insecure classification and an organized/disorganized classification. In other words, as predicted, those who were classified as preoccupied (ambivalent) and unresolved with respect to trauma (disorganized) were at greater risk for past suicidality.

Sex Differences and Attachment

The study of Adam, Keller and West (1996) was cross-sectional and did not provide information with regard to completed suicide. However, bearing in mind the limitations inherent in speculation, the authors made use of one observation from this study: Males classified as dismissing (avoidant) and not unresolved with respect to past attachment experiences were highly represented in the comparison group. This led the authors to speculate on two issues. First, that an avoidant or dismissing strategy may protect an individual from attempting suicide, through the setting aside of attachment-related or psychologically painful information. Second, since males are more likely to complete suicide, an avoidant strategy may in the long run lead an individual to greater risk of suicide through increased social isolation. These two issues regarding the relationship of a dismissing/avoidant strategy to attempted or completed suicide cannot be explained by the data at hand. Resolution depends upon prospective longitudinal studies (Adam, Keller & West, 1996).

A model of attempted suicide and completed suicide must take into account differences between males and females at across the life span. Suicidality aside for a moment, the study of Adam, West and Keller (1996) represents one of only a few attachment studies that reports a gender difference; more males were classed dismissing/avoidant in the comparison group and more females were classed as preoccupied, even though suicidal males were also highly represented in this group.

No sex differences were found in the original studies on infants (Ainsworth, et al., 1978), or reported in the initial studies with children or those first using the adult attachment interview (Main, Kaplan & Cassidy, 1985). Differences based on sex were not reported in subsequent studies using the adult attachment interview (Bakermans-Kranenburg & van Ijzendoorn, 1993).

Studies of adolescents present a somewhat different profile. For example, in non-clinical samples, some researchers report that females are more attached to peers than males (Nada Raja et al., 1992; de Jong 1992). However, others have found no differences in peer or parent attachment using the same questionnaire to assess attachment (Inventory of Parent and Peer Attachment: Greenberg et al., 1983; Armsden & Greenberg, 1987, Quintana & Lapsley, 1990). A recent meta-analysis shows males and females to differ in the relationship of attachment and self-esteem. Females' self-esteem appears more closely tied to attachment (Rice, 1990).

In one study using a new instrument, the adolescent attachment questionnaire, non-clinical, male and female adolescents scored differently on three of four sub-scales of the questionnaire (Sheldon-Keller, West, Larose & Adam, 1996). Further, clinical male and female adolescents scored differently on two of the four sub-scales, one of which was distinct from the non-clinical groups (Sheldon-Keller, West, Larose & Adam,

1996). The adolescent attachment questionnaire had good convergent validity with the adult attachment interview (Sheldon-Keller, West, Larose & Adam, 1996).

The studies noted above point to important considerations regarding the explanation of suicidality in attachment terms. Suicidal behavior is different for males and females across the life-cycle with completed suicide rates being higher for males. The male and female differences with respect to attachment are reported for adolescents but not for infants, children or adults. The reasons for this are currently unknown. Observed differences for the sexes in adolescent attachment measures may reflect a tendency for adolescents to embrace stereotypes more wholeheartedly, since gender differences are not reported in infant and child attachment behavior or with use of the adult attachment interview in adults. This may be particularly true for adolescents coming from difficult backgrounds. Less internal coherency, a diminished ability to self-regulate behaviors and affects, together with a poorly developed sense of self, may leave insecure individuals more dependent upon external social reference points to guide their thoughts and behaviors.

Summary

While attachment theory explains some very important aspects of suicidality, other social or biological factors may better account for the reasons underlying the different rates of attempted and completed suicide for males and females. This issue requires more research and the present explanation is speculative.

Demographic approaches provide considerable insight into groups at increased risk for suicide. These approaches fall short of providing insight into the dynamic nature of psychological factors psychopathology and suicidal behavior.

Family factors are most proximal to the individual at risk for suicidal behavior. Attachment research brings into sharp focus the potential of family or close personal relationships to either increase risk or provide protection from suicidality. Attachment theory provides a concise framework for understanding the development of psychopathology and suicidal behavior. Future research should attempt to examine more closely the nature of the gender differences related to attachment and perhaps provide further insight into gender differences related to suicide.

Finally, the work of Tomm (1991) characterizing the nature of healthy and pathological interpersonal patterns within the dynamic of communication within families in the context of specialized systems therapy has defined a direction for an understanding directed at a mechanism mitigating against adolescent suicidality. For example, a method for quantifying healthy and pathological interpersonal patterns of communication revealed in a retrospective case-series study that families with and without suicidality were distinguished not by the number of observed pathological interpersonal patterns. Both families with a suicidal and non-suicidal adolescent had similar rates of pathological interpersonal patterns. Rather, the groups were distinguished by a higher rate of healthy interpersonal patterns observed during interaction in therapy in families with an adolescent who was not suicidal (Lakusta, Tomm, Wilkes, & Cawthorpe, 2005).

References

Adam, K. (1990). Environmental, Psychosocial, and Psychoanalytic Aspects of Suicidal Behavior. <u>In: Suicide Over the Life Cycle: Risk Factors, Assessment, and Treatment of Suicidal Patients</u>. (Eds: S. Blumenthal & D. Kupfer). Ch. 3, pp. 39-96, American Psychiatric Press, Washington, DC.

Adam, K. (1994). Suicidal Behavior and Attachment: A Developmental Model. <u>In: Attachment in Adults: Clinical and Developmental Perspectives</u>. (Eds: M. Sperling & W. Berman) Ch. 11, pp. 275-298, Guilford Press, New York.

Adam, K. S., Sheldon-Keller, A. E., & West, M. (1996). Attachment organization and history of suicidal behavior in clinical adolescents. Journal of Consulting and Clinical Psychology, 64(2), 264–272.

Aherne, C., Coughlan, B., & Surgenor, P. (2018). Therapists' Perspectives on Suicide: A Conceptual Model of Connectedness. Psychotherapy Research : Journal of the Society for Psychotherapy Research, 28(5), 803–819. <u>https://doi.org/10.1080/10503307.2017.1359428</u>

Ainsworth, M., Blehar, M., Waters, E., & Wall, S., (1978). Patterns of attachment: A psychological study of the strange situation. Hillsdale, NJ, Erlbaum.

Alessi, N., McManus, E., Brickman, A., & Grapentine, L., (1984). Suicidal behavior among serious juvenile offenders. American Journal of Psychiatry, Vol. 141, pp. 286-287.

Armsden GC, Greenberg MT., (1987). The Inventory of Parent and Peer Attachment: Individual differences and their relationship to psychological well-being in adolescence. Journal of Youth and Adolescence, Vol. 16, pp. 427-454.

Bongar, B., (1992). Suicide: Guidelines for assessment, management and treatment. New York, Oxford University Press.

Bowlby, J., (1969). Attachment and Loss. Volume I: Attachment, New York, Basic Books.

Bowlby, J., (1973). Attachment and Loss: Volume II: Separation and Anger, New York, Basic Books.

Bowlby, J. (1977). The making and breaking of affectional bonds. II. Some principles of psychotherapy. The fiftieth Maudsley Lecture.

The British Journal of Psychiatry : The Journal of Mental Science, 130, 421–431.

Bowlby, J., (1980). Attachment and Loss. Volume III: Sadness and Depression, New York, Basic Books.

Brown, G., Harris, T., (1978). Social origins of depression: A study of psychiatric disorders in women. London, Tavistock.

Cicchetti, D., & Toth, S., (1993). Developmental perspectives on depression. Vol. 4, Rochester, University of Rochester Press.

Cicchetti, D., & Toth, S., (1995). A developmental psychopathology perspective on child abuse and neglect. Journal of the American Academy of Child and Adolescent Psychiatry, Vol. 34, pp. 541-565.

Clark, D., & Fawcett, J., (1992). Review of the risk factors for evaluation of the suicidal patient. In: Suicide: Guidelines for assessment, management and treatment. (Ed: B. Bongar) Ch. 2, pp. 16-48, New York, Oxford University Press.

Crittenden, P. (1988). Relationships at risk. In: Clinical Implications of Attachment. (Eds: J. Belskey & T. Nezworski) pp. 136-174, Hillsdale NJ, Erlbaum.

Crittenden, P., & Ainsworth, M., (1989). Child maltreatment and attachment theory. In: Child Maltreatment. (Eds: D. Cicchetti & V. Carlson) pp. 432-463, Cambridge, Cambridge University Press.

de Jong M., (1992). Attachment, individuation, and risk of suicide in late adolescence. Journal of Youth and Adolescence, Vol. 21, pp 357-373.

Edelman, G., (1987). Neural Darwinism. New York, Basic Books.

Falgares, G., Marchetti, D., De Santis, S., Carrozzino, D., Kopala-Sibley, D. C., Fulcheri, M., & Verrocchio, M. C. (2017). Attachment Styles and Suicide-Related Behaviors in Adolescence: The Mediating Role of Self-Criticism and Dependency. Frontiers in Psychiatry, 8, 36. https://doi.org/10.3389/fpsyt.2017.00036

Fonagy, P., Moran, G., & Target, M., (1993). Aggression and the psychological self. International Journal of Psychoanalysis, 74, pp. 471-485.

Fonagy, P., Steele, M., Steele, H., Moran, G., & Higgit, A., (1991). The capacity for understanding mental states: The reflective self in parent and child and its significance for security of attachment. Infant Mental Health Journal, Vol. 12, pp. 201-219.

Fraiberg, S., Adelson, E., & Shapiro, V., (1975). Ghosts in the nursery: A psychoanalytic approach to the problem of impaired infant-mother relationships. Journal of the American Academy of Child Psychiatry, Vol. 14, pp. 387-422.

Garmezy, M., (1985). Stress-resistant children: The search for protective factors. In: Recent Research in Developmental Psychopathology. (Ed: J. Stevenson) pp. 213-233, Oxford, Permagon Press.

Kovacs, M., Goldston, D., & Gastonis, C., (1993). Suicidal behaviors and childhood onset of depressive disorders: A longitudinal study. Journal of the Academy of Child and Adolescent Psychiatry, Vol. 32, 8-20.

George, C., (1994). A representational perspective of child abuse and prevention: Internal working models of attachment and caregiving. 22nd Annual Child Abuse and Neglect Symposium, May, Keystone, Colorado.

Greenberg M., Siegel J., Leitch C., (1983). The nature and importance of attachment relationships to parents and peers during adolescence. Journal of Youth and Adolescence, Vol. 12, pp. 373-386.

Lachal, J., Moro, M. R., & Spodenkiewicz, M. (2018). [An overview of suicide risk in adolescence]. Soins. Psychiatrie, 39(316), 10–13. https://doi.org/10.1016/j.spsy.2018.03.002

Lakusta C. Tomm K. Wilkes T. Cawthorpe D. (2005) A novel method for assessing interpersonal patterns of interaction in families with a suicidal adolescent. Alberta Mental Health Board Mental Health Research Showcase: Advancing through Research Innovation and Knowledge Translation. Banff Alberta Nov 28-30.

Lavigne, B., Audebert-Merilhou, E., Buisson, G., Kochman, F., Clement, J. P., & Olliac, B. (2016). [Interpersonal therapy (IPT) in child psychiatry and adolescent]. L'Encephale, 42(6), 535–539. https://doi.org/10.1016/j.encep.2015.06.009

Lester, D., (1988). The biochemical basis of suicide. Sringfield, Illinois, Charles C. Thomas.

Li, S., Galynker, I. I., Briggs, J., Duffy, M., Frechette-Hagan, A., Kim, H.-J., … Yaseen, Z. S. (2017). Attachment style and suicide behaviors in high risk psychiatric inpatients following hospital discharge: The mediating role of entrapment. Psychiatry Research, 257, 309–314. https://doi.org/10.1016/j.psychres.2017.07.072

Marvin, R., (1977). An ethological cognitive model for the attenuation of mother-child attachment behavior. In: Advances in the Study of Communication and Affect. (Eds: T. Alloway, L. Krames & P. Pliner) Vol. 3, pp. 25-60, New York, Plenum.

Marvin, R., & Greenberg, M., (1982). Preschooler's changing conceptions of their mothers: A social cognitive study of mother-child attachment. In: Children's Planning Strategies: New Directions for Child Development. No. 18, pp. 47-60, San Francisco, Josey-Bass.

Main, M, (1989). Cross-cultural studies of attachment organization: Recent studies, changing methodologies, and the concept of conditional strategies. Human Development, 33, pp. 48-61.

Main, M. (1990). Meta-cognitive knowledge, meta-cognitive monitoring, and singular (coherent) *vs.* multiple (incoherent) models of attachment. In: Attachment Across the Life Cycle. (Eds: C. Parkes, J. Stevenson-Hinde, & P. Marris, P.) Ch. 8, pp. 127-159, London, Routledge.

Main, M., & Goldwyn, R., (1991). Adult attachment classification system. Unpublished. University of California, Berkeley.

Main, M., & Hesse, E., (1990) Parent's unresolved traumatic experiences are related to infant disorganized attachment status: Is frightened and/or frightening parental behavior the linking mechanism? In: Attachment in the pre-school years. (Eds: M.
Greenberg, D. Cicchetti & R. Marvin) Ch. 5, pp. 121-183, The University of Chicago Press, Chicago.

Main, M., & Solomon, J., (1990). Procedures for identifying infants as disorganized/disoriented during the Ainsworth strange situation. In: Attachment in the preschool years. (Eds: M. Greenberg, D. Cicchetti, & E. Cummings) pp. 121-160, Chicago, University of Chicago Press.

Main, M., Kaplan, N., & Cassidy, J., (1985). Security in infancy, childhood and adulthood: A move to the level of representation. Monographs of the Society for Research in Child Development, Vol. 24, pp. 66-104.

Nada Raja, S., McGee, R., & Stanton, W., (1992). Perceived Attachment to Parents and Peers and Psychological Well-being in Adolescence. Journal of Youth and Adolescence, Vol. 21, pp. 471-485.

National Center for Health Statistics (1992). Advanced report of final mortality statistics, 1989. NCHS Monthly Vital Statistics Report, 40 (8, suppl.).

Ono, T., Tamura, R., Nishijo, H., Nakamura, K. (1993) Neural Mechanisms of recognition and memory in the limbic system. <u>In: Brain Mechanisms of Perception and Memory: From Neuron to Behavior</u> (Eds: T. Ono, L. Squire, M. Raichle, D. Perrett, M. Fukuda) pp. 330-355, Oxford, Oxford University Press.

Pennel, L., Quesada, J.-L., & Dematteis, M. (2018). Neuroticism and anxious attachment as potential vulnerability factors of repeat suicide attempts. Psychiatry Research, 264, 46–53. https://doi.org/10.1016/j.psychres.2018.03.064

Pfeffer, C., (1988). Suicidal behavior among children and adolescents: Risk identification and intervention. <u>In: American Psychiatric Press Review of Psychiatry</u>. (Eds: A. Frances & R., Hales) Vol. 7, pp. 386-402.

Quintana S., & Lapsley D., (1987). Adolescent attachment and ego identity: A structural equations approach to the continuity of adaptation. Journal of Adolescent Research, Vol. 2, pp. 393-409.

Quintana S., & Lapsley D., (1990). Rapprochement in late adolescent separation-individuation: A structural equations approach. Journal of Adolescence Vol. 13, pp. 371-385.

Rao, U., Weissman, M., Martin, J., & Hammond, R., (1993). Childhood depression and risk of suicide: A preliminary report of a longitudinal study. Journal of the American Academy of Child and Adolescent Psychiatry, Vol. 32, pp. 21-27.

Rice K., (1990). Attachment in adolescence: A narrative and meta-analytic review. Journal of Youth and Adolescence, Vol. 19, pp. 511-538.

Radke-Yarrow, M., Cummings, E. M., Kuczynski, L., & Chapman, M. (1985). Patterns of attachment in two- and three-year-olds in normal families and families with parental depression. Child Development, Vol. 56, pp. 884-893.

Ricks, M. (1985). The Social Transmission of Parental Behavior: Attachment Across Generations. In Growing Points of Attachment Theory and Research. (Eds: I., Bretherton & E. Waters) Ch. 9, pp. 211-227, Monograph of the Society for Research in Child Development.

Rutter, M., (1989). Psychosocial resilience and protective mechanisms. In: Risk and Protective Factors in the Development of Psychopathology. (Eds: J. Rolf, A Masten, D., Cicchetti, K., Nuechterlein & S. Weintraub) Ch. 9, pp. 181-214, Cambridge, Cambridge University Press.

Schneidman, E., (1992) What do Suicides have in Common? Summary of the Psychological Approach. In: Suicide: Guidelines for assessment, management and treatment. (Ed: B. Bongar) Ch. 1, pp. 3-15, New York, Oxford University Press.

Seymour, S., (1990) Genetic Factors in suicide: Family, twin, and adoption studies. In: Suicide Over the Life Cycle: Risk Factors, Assessment, and Treatment of Suicidal Patients. (Eds: S. Blumenthal & D. Kupfer). Ch. 5, pp. 127-134, American Psychiatric Press, Washington, DC.

Sheftall, A. H., Mathias, C. W., Furr, R. M., & Dougherty, D. M. (2013). Adolescent attachment security, family functioning, and suicide attempts. Attachment & Human Development, 15(4), 368–383. https://doi.org/10.1080/14616734.2013.782649

Sokol, M., & Pfeffer, C., (1992). Suicidal behavior of children. In: Suicide: Guidelines for assessment, management and treatment. (Ed: B. Bongar) Ch. 4, pp. 69-83, New York, Oxford University Press.

Sroufe, L. (1983). Infant-caregiver attachment and patterns of maladaptation in preschool: The role of maladaptation and competence. In: Minnesota symposium of child psychology.

(Eds: M. Perlmutter) Vol. 16, pp. 41-81. Minneapolis, University of Minnesota Press.

Sroufe, A., (1988). The role of infant-caregiver attachment in development. In: Clinical Implications of Attachment. (Eds: J. Belskey & T. Nezworski) pp. 18-41, Hillsdale, NJ, Erlbaum.

Sroufe, A., & Fleeson, J., (1986). Attachment and the construction of relationships. In: The Nature and Development of Relationships. (Eds: W. Hartup & Z. Rubin) pp. 51-71, Hillsdale, NJ, Erlbaum.

Sroufe, A., Waters, E., (1977). Attachment as an Organizational Construct. Child Development, 48, pp. 1184-1199.

Stern, D., (1985). The interpersonal world of the infant. New York, Basic Books.

Tomm, KM. (1991). Beginnings of a "HIPs and PIPs" approach to psychiatric assessment. The Calgary Participator, 1 (2): 21-24.

Tucker, D.M. (1992) Devloping emotions and cortical networks. In: Developmental behavioral neuroscience; The Minnesota symposia on child psychology, (Ed: M. Gunnar & C. Nelson) Volume 24, pp. 74-128, Erlbaum, Hilsdale, N.J.

Vallant, G., & Blumenthal, S., (1990). Suicide over the life cycle: Risk factors and life-span development. <u>In: Suicide Over the Life Cycle: Risk Factors, Assessment, and Treatment of Suicidal Patients</u>. (Eds: S. Blumenthal & D. Kupfer). Ch. 1, pp. 1-16, American Psychiatric Press, Washington, DC.

West, M., & Keller, A., (1994). Patterns of Relating: An Adult Attachment Perspective. New York, Guilford.

Zahn-Waxler, C., Cummings, E. M., Iannotti, R. J., & Radke-Yarrow, M. (1984). Young children of depressed parents: A population at risk for affective problems. In D. Cicchetti, & K. Schneider-Rosen (Eds.), Childhood Depression (pp. 81-105). San Francisco: Jossey-Bass.

Zisk, A., Abbott, C. H., Ewing, S. K., Diamond, G. S., & Kobak, R. (2017). The Suicide Narrative Interview: adolescents' attachment expectancies and symptom severity in a clinical sample. Attachment & Human Development, 19(5), 447–462. https://doi.org/10.1080/14616734.2016.1269234

www.ingramcontent.com/pod-product-compliance
Lightning Source LLC
Chambersburg PA
CBHW020455220526
45464CB00002B/992